SIMPLE COLON
DIET COOKBOOK

A Healthy Colon Keeps the Sickness Away.

By

CYNTHIA LEONARD

TABLE OF CONTENTS

INTRODUCTION: Understanding the Colon Diet

What is A Colon Diet?

Although there isn't a single "colon diet" per se, there are dietary suggestions and considerations for preserving a healthy colon and avoiding colon-related health concerns including colon cancer and digestive disorders. The main goals of these dietary suggestions are to improve colon health and lower the risk of colon-related disorders. The following food recommendations may help maintain a healthy colon:

High-Fibre Foods: Fibre-rich diets are often advised for colon health. Constipation may be avoided by consuming enough fibre, which encourages regular bowel motions. Additionally, colon cancer risk may be reduced. Fruits, vegetables, whole grains, legumes and nuts are good sources of dietary fibre.

Fruits and Vegetables: Including a variety of fruits and vegetables in your diet will help you obtain the fibre, antioxidants, and vitamins and minerals you need to maintain good colon health. To receive a variety of nutrients, aim for a colourful blend.

Whole Grains: Wherever feasible, go for whole grains instead than processed ones. Oats, whole wheat bread and other whole grains provide higher fibre and minerals that may help maintain digestive health.

Limit Red and Processed Meats: Studies have linked a high intake of red and processed meats, such as bacon, sausage and hot dogs, to an increased risk of colon cancer. Limiting these meals and choosing lean protein sources instead, such as chicken, fish and plant-based proteins, is a smart choice.

Foods that have been fermented with probiotics: Probiotics are good bacteria that help improve intestinal health. A healthy gut microbiota may be maintained by eating probiotic-rich foods including yoghurt, kefir, sauerkraut and kimchi.

Water intake: Maintaining a healthy water intake is crucial for digestive health in general. Water aids in the digestion process' smooth operation and softens stools.

Limit Your Alcohol and Tobacco Use: Alcohol and tobacco use have been related to an elevated risk of colon cancer. It may be good for your colon and general health to cut down on or stop these practices.

Control your portions: Overeating and obesity might raise your chance of developing colon cancer. This risk may be reduced by eating healthfully and engaging in frequent physical exercise.

While food has an impact on colon health, routine screening procedures like colonoscopies are essential for the early identification and prevention of colon cancer. If you have a family history of colon cancer or other risk factors, talk to your healthcare professional about your screening schedule.

It's important to note that everyone has different nutritional demands, so it's a good idea to speak with a healthcare provider or a qualified dietitian to develop a customised eating plan that suits your unique health requirements. Also for best outcomes, a balanced diet should be paired with other healthy lifestyle decisions like regular exercise and quitting smoking. A balanced diet is only one part of total colon health.

Importance Of A Healthy Colon

The large intestine, sometimes referred to as the colon, is essential to sustaining general health and wellbeing. Having a healthy colon is important for the following reasons:

Digestive Function: The colon is in charge of producing and eliminating faeces as well as absorbing water and electrolytes. It assists in maintaining the body's electrolyte balance and optimum hydration while removing waste. Effective digestion is ensured by a healthy colon, which also guards against constipation and diarrhoea.

Nutrients Absorption: The colon also contributes to the absorption of certain nutrients, such as vitamins produced by gut bacteria *(such as vitamin K and several B vitamins)*. The best absorption of nutrients is facilitated by a healthy colon.

Gut Health: The gut microbiota, a huge colony of helpful bacteria, lives in the colon. These microorganisms create crucial nutrients, aid in the digestion of undigested food, and strengthen the immune system. Better general health is connected with a gut microbiota that is balanced and diversified, which is supported by a healthy colon.

Support for the Immune System: The gut is home to a significant percentage of the body's immune system. An immune system that is robust and balanced is influenced by gut health. When the colon is working properly, it aids in stopping dangerous microorganisms from infecting the body and entering the bloodstream.

Removal of Toxins: The colon acts as a filter to eliminate toxins and waste from the body. A healthy colon effectively removes waste, lowering the chance that toxins may be reabsorbed into the circulation and cause negative health consequences.

Disease Prevention: Keeping your colon healthy helps lower your chance of developing a number of gastrointestinal diseases, such as diverticulitis, diverticular disease and irritable bowel syndrome *(IBS)*. Regular exams, including colonoscopies, may help identify any problems early on when they are easier to treat.

Overall Health: Overall health and colon health are strongly related. Constipation or diarrhoea that persists over time may have a detrimental effect on a person's quality of life. You may improve your entire physical and mental health by encouraging a healthy colon.

Adopt a fibre-rich, balanced diet, remain hydrated, exercise often and abstain from behaviours that might damage the digestive system, such as smoking and binge drinking, in order to maintain a healthy colon.

How this Cookbook Can Help You

For those seeking to enhance their digestive health and general well-being, this "Colon Diet Cookbook" will be a valuable resource. By collecting water and nutrients from digested food and removing waste, the colon, commonly referred to as the large intestine, serves an important function in the digestive system. Digestion and general health depend on keeping the colon in good shape. Benefits from a colon diet cookbook are as follows:

Promotes Digestive Health: Easy-to-digest and soft on the colon foods are often included in the dishes in a colon diet cookbook. Constipation, diarrhoea and bloating are just a few of the digestive problems that these dishes may treat.

Promotes a High-fibre Diet: Fibre is crucial for keeping the colon healthy. Recipes that are high in fibre from fruits, vegetables, whole grains and legumes may be found in many cookbooks for the colon cleanse. Fibre lowers the incidence of colon-related disorders and aids in the promotion of regular bowel motions.

Reduces Processed Foods: The health of the colon may be harmed by processed and highly processed foods. Cookbooks for the colon diet often place an emphasis on whole, unprocessed products and advise against eating processed meals since they frequently include chemicals and preservatives that might aggravate the colon.

A Colon Diet Cookbook normally places a strong emphasis on providing balanced nourishment. It could have meals that contain a range of the vitamins, minerals and nutrients essential for good health generally, including foods that support the gut microbiota.

Weight management: It's crucial for colon health to maintain a healthy weight. A cookbook for the colon diet could include dishes that are good for controlling weight, which can lower the risk of illnesses connected to the colon, such as colorectal cancer.

Colorectal cancer prevention: A greater risk of colorectal cancer has been associated with several dietary variables. A cookbook for the colon diet could include dishes that include ingredients high in antioxidants, vitamins and minerals, which are thought to have cancer-preventing effects.

Education and Awareness: A lot of cookbooks for the colon diet include information on the value of colon health, typical digestive problems and maintenance advice. People may use this knowledge to make educated eating decisions.

Meal Planning and Variety: It's important to have a varied diet for general wellness. You may find a variety of recipes in a colon diet cookbook to assist you in creating well-balanced meals and avoiding dietary boredom.

Supports Specific disorders: Some colon diet cookbooks may provide recipes that are adapted to the dietary requirements of people with certain disorders, such as irritable bowel syndrome (IBS) or Crohn's disease.

Inspiration for Cooking: Trying out new dishes may be enjoyable and motivating. You may learn fun and tasty ways to add colon-friendly items to your diet from a cookbook dedicated to the diet.

Chapter 1: Getting Started

Kitchen Essentials for the Colon Diet

A colon-healthy diet often emphasises items that support a healthy digestive system and lower the risk of colorectal issues. Although there are no certain kitchen necessities that are just appropriate for a "**colon diet**," you may fill your kitchen with products that promote general digestive health. Few kitchen necessities for a diet that's good for your colon are:

Foods high in fibre are necessary for encouraging regular bowel motions and sustaining colon health. Oats, brown rice, quinoa, beans, lentils and other healthful grains, fruits, and vegetables should all be in plenty.

Leafy Greens: Vegetables like spinach, kale and Swiss chard are a great source of fibre, vitamins and minerals that are good for your digestive system.

Probiotic-rich foods: Probiotics assist in maintaining a balanced population of gut flora. Be sure to eat fermented foods like yoghurt, kefir, kimchi, sauerkraut and others.

Lean Protein: Include lean protein-rich foods including tofu, fish and skinless chicken. These are less difficult to digest than fatty meats.

Olive oil, avocados and almonds are sources of healthful fats that promote digestive health.

Herbs & spices: Ginger, turmeric, mint and fennel may reduce inflammation and pain in the digestive system.

Fruits Whole: Always have a selection of fresh fruits on hand. Fruits that are especially good for your colon are apples, pears, berries and citrus fruits.

Natural Sweeteners: Choose unrefined sweeteners like honey or maple syrup over artificial sweeteners.

Whole-Grain Flours: If you like baking, consider using whole-grain flours like whole wheat, oat or almond for a more nutritious take on your go-to recipes.

Almonds, walnuts, flaxseeds and chia seeds are great sources of fibre and good fats.

Whole-grain pasta and bread are excellent choices if you want to boost your intake of fibre.

Low-Sodium Broth: For stews and soups, use low-sodium chicken or vegetable broth.

Tea: Herbal infusions with digestive easing properties, such as peppermint and ginger, are available.

Water: Maintaining enough hydration is important for intestinal health in general.

Purchase storage containers for leftovers and ingredients for meals to save time and prevent food waste.

Tools for the kitchen: A food processor for slicing vegetables, a steamer for cooking vegetables without destroying their nutrients and a blender for smoothies may all be useful.

Cutting boards and knives: Making meals is made simpler and safer with high-quality cutting boards and razor-sharp blades.

Mason jars are particularly helpful for preserving homemade condiments, dressings and overnight oats.

Use nonstick, stainless steel or cast iron cookware if you want to cook healthily since these materials use less oil.

Food Labels: Become familiar with food labels to make educated decisions regarding packaged foods.

Tips for Success And Common Misconceptions

It might be beneficial to use a colon diet cookbook to support good digestion and general health. You should be aware of several widespread misunderstandings about nutrition and colon health, however. Here are some guidelines for achievement and debunking such myths:

Success Strategies:

Consult a Healthcare Professional: It's crucial to speak with a qualified dietitian or a healthcare provider before making any big dietary changes, particularly if you have certain digestive issues or medical illnesses. They may provide you customised advice and make sure your food choices support your health objectives.

Pick a Reliable Cookbook: When choosing a cookbook for a colon cleanse, search for trustworthy publications produced by dietitians, nutritionists or healthcare experts. Make sure the recipes support digestive health and are based on scientific research.

A diet high in fibre helps support a healthy digestive system and regular bowel motions. Include a range of high-fibre foods in your meals, such as fruits, vegetables, whole grains, legumes and nuts.

Keep Hydrated: Proper hydration is essential for maintaining gut health. To aid in softening stools and stave against constipation, drink lots of water throughout the day.

Foods containing Probiotics, such as yoghurt, kefir, sauerkraut, and kimchi, may help maintain a balanced gut microbiota. Include them in your diet to encourage healthy gut flora.

Limit Processed foods since they may harm your gut's health. Limit your consumption of processed foods, fast food and sugary snacks.

Portion control is important since eating too much might strain your digestive system. To prevent pain and stomach problems, pay attention to portion quantities.

Eat Slowly: Digestive pain might result from eating too rapidly. To promote digestion, chew your food completely and take your time eating.

Common Misunderstandings:

Extreme detox diets or colon cleanses are erroneously believed to be essential for a healthy colon. The truth is that your body has built-in detoxification processes, therefore severe diets may really be damaging.

Avoid following trendy eating plans that promise rapid cures for colon health. Dietary adjustments that can be maintained over time are more beneficial.

Enemas and colonics: Some individuals think that enemas and colonics are crucial for colon health. When essential for certain medical circumstances, these treatments should only be carried out under physician supervision.

One-Size-Fits-All Everybody has a different digestive system. Don't assume that everyone will have the same results from a certain colon diet. Adapt your diet to your own requirements and tastes.

Neglecting Whole Foods: might be ineffective to rely entirely on supplements or certain foods for colon health while excluding a balanced diet rich in whole foods.

Holistic health encompasses more than just your gut. The maintenance of intestinal health requires a balanced diet, frequent exercise, stress reduction and enough sleep.

Chapter 2: RECIPES - Cleansing Starters

A. Menu To Revitalise Your Mornings

Lemon and Ginger Detox Elixir:

A well-liked beverage known as lemon and ginger detox elixir is touted as having cleansing and health-improving properties. You might try the following easy recipe:

Ingredients:

- Fresh ginger root, 1 to 2 inches long, peeled, grated or thinly sliced
- Juiced lemons, 1 to 2
- 1-2 teaspoons of raw honey, tasted before using.
- 2 cups of ideally filtered water
- You may add a dash of ground turmeric or a sprinkle of cayenne pepper for flavour and health benefits.

Instructions:

Water on the Boil: Begin by bringing the two cups of water to a boil. For this, you may use a saucepan or a kettle.

Prepare the ginger by peeling, grating or slicing it while the water is heating. This elixir's main component, ginger, is known for its flavour and purifying effects.

Ginger and Water: Once the water is at a rolling boil, add the ginger. Allow it to boil for five to ten minutes on low heat. Ginger's flavours and healthy ingredients will be released into the water with the aid of simmering.

After simmering, drain the mixture to get rid of the ginger by pouring it into a cup or another heat-resistant vessel. A tea infuser or a fine-mesh strainer are both acceptable.

Lemon Juice: Add the juice of a couple of lemons to the ginger-infused water. Depending on your preferred flavour, adjust the quantity of lemon juice. Lemon has a light citrus flavour and is a good source of vitamin C.

Add 1-2 teaspoons of raw honey to the liquid and whisk until the honey is dissolved. Depending on the sweetness you choose, adjust the honey quantity. Honey has extra health advantages in addition to its ability to sweeten food.

Add a dash of ground turmeric or a sprinkle of cayenne pepper, if desired, for additional detoxification power. These components are said to have cleansing qualities and may give the elixir a distinctive flavour.

Enjoy: Drink this warm detox elixir made with lemon and ginger. It may be had all day as a pleasant beverage or first thing in the morning on an empty stomach.

While this elixir is a popular option for cleansing and fostering general well-being, keep in mind that for maximum health, a balanced diet and way of life are necessary.

Green Smoothie Bowl:

A wholesome and scrumptious way to start your day is with a green smoothie bowl. The following is a simple recipe that you may change to your taste:

Ingredients:

Applied to the smoothie bowl:

- 2 frozen, ripe bananas
- 1 cup fresh or frozen spinach or kale leaves
- 12 an avocado
- Greek yoghurt in the amount of half a cup, or a dairy-free substitute like almond yoghurt
- *(Dairy or dairy-free)* 1/2 cup milk
- 1 tablespoon of optionally sweetened honey or maple syrup
- 0.5 teaspoons of optional vanilla extract
- For the toppings *(which you may personalise)*
- Sliced strawberries Sliced kiwi
- Chia seed
- Seed hemp
- Granola
- Almonds, sliced
- Flakes of coconut
- Vibrant berries
- Chopped banana
- For drizzling, use honey or maple syrup

Instructions:

Put together your toppings:

The fruits you'll be using as toppings should be washed and sliced.

If you want to add seeds, nuts or granola, measure them out beforehand. Make and blend the smoothie:

Blend the milk, Greek yoghurt, frozen bananas, spinach or kale, avocado, honey, maple syrup or vanilla extract if desired.

Blend the ingredients until it's creamy and smooth. You may add a bit of extra milk if it's too thick to get the consistency you want.

Build the Bowl:

In a bowl, pour the green smoothie.

Put on toppings:

Place the toppings of your choice on top of the smoothie. Make it aesthetically attractive and imaginative.

Serve and Take Note:

Get a spoon and start eating! As you eat, mix the toppings into the smoothie for a variety of flavours and textures.

Feel free to add other ingredients to your green smoothie bowl, such as flax seeds, spirulina or various kinds of fruits and vegetables, to suit your taste and dietary needs.

Berry Cleansing Blast:

A berry cleansing blast is a tasty and nourishing smoothie that may aid in bodily detoxification and rehydration. Here is a simple recipe you might try:

Ingredients:

- 1 cup of mixed berries, including blackberries, raspberries, blueberries and strawberries.
- To add more greens, use 1/2 cup of spinach or kale leaves.
- 1/2 cup of unsweetened coconut water or almond milk.
- Greek yoghurt or dairy-free yoghurt, *optionally*, in the amount of 1/2 cup.
- Chia seeds, one tablespoon, **optional** *(for extra fibre and omega-3 fatty acids)*.
- 1 teaspoon of optionally sweetening honey or maple syrup

- Ice cubes *(optional, for a smoothie that is cooler)*.

Instructions:

Thoroughly wash all the berries and leaves.

Blend the mixed berries, spinach or kale, almond milk or coconut water, Greek yoghurt *(if used)*, chia seeds *(if using)*, honey or maple syrup *(if using)* and any other ingredients into a smooth smoothie.

You may also add a few ice cubes if you want your smoothie to be cooler and thicker.

The mixture should be smooth and creamy after blending all the components. To make sure everything is well blended, you may need to pause and scrape down the sides of the blender.

Taste the smoothie and, *if required*, add additional honey or maple syrup to increase the sweetness.

Fill a glass with the Berry Cleansing Blast, top with more berries or chia seeds as desired and serve right away.

The berries and greens in this hydrating smoothie are a rich source of minerals, vitamins and antioxidants. It's a terrific option for a nutritious breakfast or snack that can help your body's natural detoxification processes get started in the morning.

B. Gut-Friendly Snacks

Probiotic Yogurt Parfait:

A probiotic yoghurt parfait blends the healthiness of yoghurt with the sweetness of fruit and the crunch of oats for a delectable and nutritious treat. Yoghurt is a fantastic source of probiotics, which are good bacteria that support intestinal health. Simple recipe for probiotic yoghurt parfait:

Ingredients:

- 1 cup of yoghurt, either Greek or another kind.
- 1/2 cup of granola, either homemade or purchased.
- Strawberries, blueberries, and raspberries make up half a Cup of the mixed berries.
- 1 tablespoon of optionally additional honey for sweetness
- Vanilla extract, 1/4 teaspoon, **optional** *(for flavour)*.

Instructions:

Prepare your ingredients beforehand. If necessary, slice any bigger berries after washing the others.

Mix the honey and vanilla essence into the yoghurt to give your parfait a hint of sweetness. Depending on your preferred level of sweetness, adjust the honey. If you like your parfait without additional sweets, you may easily omit this step.

Choose a transparent bowl or glass that has a large aperture to highlight the layers. Yoghurt should first be layered into the glass's bottom.

After that, sprinkle oats over the yoghurt. You may use the granola of your choice, whether it is plain, honey-sweetened or comes in a unique flavour.

Over the granola, now put a layer of mixed berries. To give your parfait colour and flavour, use a variety of fruit. Use your imagination while coming up with combos.

Repeat the procedure of stacking, beginning with a fresh layer of yoghurt and finishing with granola and berries. Three layers are a frequent option, but you may construct as many as you wish.

Add a final dollop of yoghurt to the top of your parfait and decorate with more berries and granola for texture.

Add more honey on top if you'd like for added sweetness and appearance.

Instantaneously serve your probiotic yoghurt parfait as a balanced breakfast, snack, or dessert. Enjoy!

You are welcome to add other fruits, nuts, seeds or even a dash of cinnamon to your yoghurt parfait to enhance flavour and nutrients. This recipe is quite flexible in terms of your dietary needs and taste preferences.

Cucumber and Hummus Bites:
Bites of cucumber and hummus make an easy and nutritious starter or snack. They are simple to prepare and excellent as a light snack or for gatherings. An easy recipe for bite-sized cucumber and hummus:

Ingredients:

- One cucumber
- 1 cup of the hummus of your choice
- Cherry tomatoes may be used as a garnish.
- Fresh dill or parsley is optional as a garnish.
- *Optional* olive oil for drizzling
- Pepper and salt as desired

Instructions:

Cucumber should be well washed and then sliced into pieces that are each approximately 1/2 inch thick. Peeling the cucumber is optional if you like a more elegant appearance.

Use a fork to delicately score each cucumber slice's top in a crisscross pattern if you want to add a decorative design. Although *optional*, this step adds a pleasant touch.

Each cucumber slice should have a large dab of hummus on it. To make it neater, use a spoon or a piping bag.

The cucumber and hummus bits may optionally be topped with chopped cherry tomatoes, a drizzle of olive oil, fresh parsley or dill. These decorations give the bites flavour and aesthetic appeal.

Add a dash of salt and pepper to taste the bits. Hummus may be pretty salty on its own, so be careful with the salt.

Serve the cucumber and hummus bits right away after placing them on a serving plate. Although they may be briefly chilled before serving, they are at their finest when they are still fresh.

Tips and Variations:

To change up the flavour of your bites, experiment with several hummus flavours, such as traditional, roasted red pepper or garlic hummus.

For added flavour, think about sprinkling over some paprika, red pepper flakes or za'atar spice.

As a substitute for the cucumber, you may alternatively use bell pepper or zucchini pieces that are crisp.

For the greatest flavour and texture, keep any leftover cucumber and hummus bits in the refrigerator and eat them within a day or two.

Bites of cucumber and hummus are adaptable and may be made to your preferences.

Gut-Healing Bone Broth:

A nourishing and calming beverage that may help improve gut health and provide a number of other health advantages is gut-healing bone broth. The nutrients and collagen from the bones are extracted by boiling vegetables, herbs and bones for a long time. Recipe for bone broth that helps the digestive system:

Ingredients:

Bones: A variety of bones, including those from chicken, cattle, hog and even fish, may be used. Joint bones and bones with marrow are particularly advantageous. Try to get two to three pounds of bones.

1-2 celery stalks, 2-3 carrots, 1-2 onions and a couple garlic cloves, all coarsely diced.

Fresh herbs: A few fresh bay leaves, thyme and parsley.

2 teaspoons of apple cider vinegar. This facilitates the bones' mineral extraction.

Water: About 10 to 12 cups should be plenty to completely cover all the ingredients in your saucepan.

To taste, add salt and pepper.

Optional Supplements for Additional Nutrients:

Ginger: A thinly sliced, fresh piece of ginger.

A tiny piece of fresh turmeric root or one teaspoon of powdered turmeric.

A little quantity of dried shiitake or other therapeutic mushrooms.

A slice of kombu or other sea vegetables for extra nutrients
is considered seaweed.

Instructions:

Heat the oven to 350°F (175°C) before roasting the bones.
Roast the bones for 30 to 45 minutes after placing them on a
baking sheet. Although **optional**, this step might improve the
flavour of your broth.

Combine ingredients: Place the roasted bones (*if using*), veggies,
herbs, apple cider vinegar and any other ingredients in a
large stockpot or slow cooker.

Add Water: Fill the saucepan with enough water to cover all
the ingredients.

Simmer: After the mixture comes to a boil, turn the heat
down to low and let the mixture to simmer. While beef or
hog broth may need 12–24 hours to boil, chicken broth
should simmer for at least 8–12 hours. More nutrients are
extracted when food is simmered for longer.

Skim the Foam: After simmering for the first hour or so, foam may start to appear on the surface. With a spoon, skim it off and throw it away.

After the broth has simmered to your liking, strain it to get rid of the particles into a big basin or container using a fine-mesh screen or cheesecloth.

Season the broth to taste with salt and pepper. Start with one teaspoon of salt and then titrate to your taste.

Allow the broth to cool to room temperature before storing it in the refrigerator or freezer in portion-controlled bags for later use.

Enjoy your gut-healing bone broth as a warm beverage, as a foundation for soups and stews or by adding it to other dishes. A daily cup of bone broth may promote intestinal health and provide important minerals.

Chapter 3: Fibre-Packed Meals

A. Breakfast Boosters

Quinoa and Chia Porridge:

A substantial and healthy breakfast choice that is high in protein, fibre and vital elements is quinoa and chia porridge. Here is a simple recipe you might try:

Ingredients:

- 0.5 cups of quinoa
- Chia seeds, 2 teaspoons
- 2 cups of your preferred milk, such as almond milk
- 1 to 2 tablespoons of honey or maple syrup (adjust to taste)
- One-half teaspoon of vanilla extract
- 1/8 teaspoon cinnamon powder
- Add a little salt
- Your preferred toppings, such as fresh berries, sliced bananas, almonds, seeds and coconut flakes

Instructions:

Under cold running water, thoroughly rinse the quinoa. By doing this, any bitter saponins are removed. Flow freely.

Quinoa that has been washed and chia seeds go together in a medium pot.

To the pot, add the almond milk, maple syrup *(or honey)*, vanilla bean paste, ground cinnamon and a dash of salt. The items should be stirred together.

Bring the mixture to a boil in the saucepan over medium-high heat.

Once it starts to boil, turn down the heat and cover the pan. Stirring periodically, simmer for 15 to 20 minutes or until the quinoa is cooked and the stew has thickened.

You may add a little extra milk to the mixture to get the proper consistency if it thickens up too much before the quinoa is finished cooking.

Remove the skillet from the heat when the quinoa is done and the porridge is creamy.

If required, taste the porridge and adjust the sweetness or spices.

Assemble bowls of the quinoa and chia porridge and top with your preferred garnishes. Among the best choices are fresh berries, banana slices, almonds, seeds and coconut flakes.

While it's still warm, serve your wonderful and healthy quinoa and chia porridge.

Avocado and Black Bean Breakfast Tacos:
Breakfast tacos with avocado and black beans are a tasty and healthy way to start the day. In this dish, black beans and avocado are combined with the protein and fibre of black beans and are all wrapped in a warm tortilla. You may add your own toppings and spices to these tacos to make them your own. Here is a simple recipe to get you going:

Ingredients:

Regarding the filling of avocado and black beans:
1 avocado, mashed or cut into slices.

1 can (15 oz) washed and drained black beans

1/2 red onion, chopped finely

1 diced red, yellow or green bell pepper

1-2 minced garlic cloves

1 teaspoon of cumin, ground

Pepper and salt as desired

Cooking with olive oil

Putting together tacos:
4-6 tiny tortillas, either flour or corn, as desired

Four big eggs

Choose from cheddar, Monterey Jack or 1/2 cup of other shredded cheese.

(Optional toppings) Sour cream, salsa or spicy sauce

Leafy fresh cilantro is optional as a garnish.

(Optional for serving) Lime wedges

Instructions:

Filling with avocado and black beans: One tablespoon of olive oil is heated over medium heat in a big skillet.

Add the bell pepper and red onion, chop them, and sauté for 3 to 4 minutes or until they start to soften.

Add the ground cumin and minced garlic, stir and cook for a further one to two minutes until fragrant.

To the skillet, add the rinsed and drained black beans. Cook for a further 2 to 3 minutes while partially mashing the beans with a fork or potato masher. This will aid in giving the filling a creamy texture.

To taste, add salt and pepper to the food.

Get the tortillas ready: The tortillas should be warmed and malleable by heating them in a dry pan over medium heat for 20 to 30 seconds on each side or by placing them in a moist paper towel and heating them in the microwave for 20 to 30 seconds.

Prepare the eggs:
A little additional olive oil should be heated over medium heat in a different skillet. In the skillet, crack the eggs and fry them to your preferred doneness *(scrambled, fried or sunny-side-up)*.

Build the tacos: On a spotless surface, spread out the heated tortillas. Each tortilla should have mashed avocado on it.

Spread the avocado with the black bean mixture then add scrambled eggs and cheese on top.

Serve and garnish: Salsa, spicy sauce, sour cream and fresh cilantro leaves are optional garnishes.

For an additional flavour boost, serve lime wedges with the avocado and black bean breakfast tacos.

Oatmeal with Mixed Berries:

Ingredients:

- Rolled oats, 1 cup
- 2 cups of milk *(cow, almond or oat milks are all acceptable types of milk)*.
- 0.5 teaspoons of optional vanilla extract
- 1 tablespoon of optionally sweetened honey or maple syrup.

- Strawberries, blueberries, raspberries or blackberries make up one cup of mixed berries.
- *(Optional)* 1/4 cup chopped nuts, such as almonds, walnuts or pecans.
- Add a little salt

Instructions:

The mixed berries should be rinsed and placed aside. Depending on what's available, you may use fresh or frozen berries.

Mix the milk, rolled oats and a dash of salt in a medium saucepan. You may also add honey or maple syrup at this point if you want to add some sweetness. To blend, thoroughly stir.

Bring the mixture to a simmer in the saucepan over medium heat. For around 5-7 minutes or when the oats are creamy and have absorbed the majority of the liquid, reduce the heat to low and stir periodically.
Cook a little longer if you want a thicker consistency; if it becomes too thick, add a little more milk.

Remove the pot from the heat when the oats are cooked to the desired consistency. Add vanilla extract for flavour if you'd like.

Muesli should be divided into serving dishes.

If using, add chopped nuts and mixed berries on top of the muesli.

If you want additional sweetness, you may also add a bit more honey or maple syrup on top.

Enjoy a filling and healthy breakfast by serving heated muesli with mixed berries!

B. Satisfying Lunches

Roasted Vegetable Quinoa Bowl:

Here is a great dish for a Quinoa Bowl with Roasted Vegetables. This rich, nutritious meal is bursting with flavour. You may add your own veggies and toppings to it.

Ingredients:

Regarding the roasted veggies:

- 2 cups of assorted veggies, diced into bite-sized pieces, such as bell peppers, zucchini, cherry tomatoes, broccoli and carrots.
- Olive oil, two teaspoons
- One tablespoon of dried thyme
- 1 teaspoon of rosemary, dry
- Pepper and salt as desired

Regarding the quinoa:

- 1 cup of rinsed and drained quinoa
- 2 cups of water or vegetable broth
- Salt as desired

To be Dressed:

- Olive oil, 3 tablespoons
- Balsamic vinegar, two teaspoons
- 1 minced garlic clove
- Dijon mustard, 1 teaspoon
- Pepper and salt as desired
- *(Optional)* For toppings
- Crumbled feta cheese
- Slivered almonds, chopped pine nuts or fresh basil leaves.
- Sliced avocados.

- Flakes of red pepper *(for a little heat)*.

Instructions:

Turn on the oven to 425 °F (220 °C).

The chopped veggies, olive oil, dried thyme, dried rosemary, salt and pepper should all be combined in a large mixing dish. To uniformly coat the veggies, combine everything and toss.

On a baking sheet covered with parchment paper or a silicone baking mat, spread out the seasoned veggies in a single layer.

The veggies should be roasted in a preheated oven for 20 to 25 minutes, or until they are soft and just beginning to caramelise. Stirring the vegetables halfway through will help to ensure equal cooking. Take out of the oven, then place aside.

Use a fine-mesh strainer to thoroughly rinse the quinoa under cold water while the veggies are roasting. Quinoa

that has been washed, vegetable broth (*or water*) and a dash of
salt should all be combined in a medium pot.

Bring to a boil, then lower the heat to a simmer, cover the
pan and cook the quinoa for approximately 15 minutes, or
until the liquid is absorbed. With a fork, fluff the quinoa
and let it gently cool.

To create the dressing, combine the olive oil, balsamic
vinegar, garlic powder, Dijon mustard, salt and pepper in a
small bowl.

Divide the cooked quinoa among serving dishes to
construct the bowls. Add some of the roasted veggies to the
top of each bowl.

On top of the quinoa and veggies, drizzle the dressing.

Add your preferred garnishes, such as avocado slices, feta
cheese crumbles, fresh basil, pine nuts or slivered almonds,
and a dash of red pepper flakes for spice. Serve.

Lentil and Kale Salad:

A tasty and healthy recipe that is loaded with protein, fibre and minerals is lentil and kale salad. Here is a simple recipe you might try:

Ingredients:

To make the salad:
- 1 cup of drained and washed green or brown lentils
- Water in 4 glasses
- Remove the stems from 1 bunch of kale and slice the leaves into bite-sized pieces.
- 1 chopped red bell pepper
- 1/2 red onion, chopped finely
- Half a cup of cherry tomatoes
- (*Optional*) 1/4 cup feta cheese
- 14 cup finely chopped fresh parsley
- To taste, add salt and black pepper.

When dressing:
- Extra virgin olive oil, 1/4 cup
- 2 tablespoons (*or around 1 lemon*) of lemon juice
- 2 minced garlic cloves
- Dijon mustard, 1 teaspoon

- 1 teaspoon of optionally sweetened honey or maple syrup
- To taste, add salt and black pepper.

Instructions:
Lentil preparation:

Combine the washed lentils with 4 cups of water in a medium saucepan.

When the lentils are cooked but still firm, cook for 20 to 25 minutes at a simmer after bringing to a boil. They shouldn't be mushy. Let the lentils cool after draining any extra water.

The kale, as follows: Add the chopped kale to a large mixing bowl then for a few minutes, massage some salt and a little olive oil into the kale until it is soft and just beginning to wilt. It will become more delicious and less rough as a result.

Creating the dressing: Olive oil, lemon juice, chopped garlic, Dijon mustard, honey _(if used)_, salt and black pepper should all be well mixed in a small bowl.

Putting the salad together: To the dish containing the massaged kale, add the cooked lentils, diced red bell pepper, sliced red onion and half of the cherry tomatoes.

When everything is well coated, drizzle the dressing over the salad and toss to combine.

For more flavour and garnish, you may top with crumbled feta cheese and chopped fresh parsley.

If necessary, add extra salt, pepper or lemon juice after tasting the salad. Before serving, let the salad rest for 10 to 15 minutes to let the flavours blend.

This lentil and kale salad works well as a side dish or as the main course for a light lunch or supper. It's a terrific addition to your cuisine since it's tasty and healthful.

Sweet Potato and Black Bean Burrito Bowl:

As it blends the flavours of roasted sweet potatoes, black beans and a variety of toppings, this dish is not only delicious but also nutrient-dense. Feel free to alter it as you choose.

Ingredients:

Regarding the sweet potatoes:
- Peeled and sliced into bite-sized chunks, two medium sweet potatoes.
- Olive oil, two teaspoons.
- One tablespoon of chilli powder.
- 1/8 teaspoon cumin powder,
- Pepper and salt as desired.

Regarding the black beans:
- 1 can (15 ounces) rinsed and drained black beans
- 1 minced garlic clove
- 1/8 teaspoon cumin powder
- 50 ml of chilli powder
- Pepper and salt as desired

To make the salsa:
- Diced tomatoes, 1 cup
- 1/2 cup red onion, chopped
- 14 cup finely minced fresh cilantro
- 1 lime's juice
- To taste, add salt and pepper for assembly.
- Cooked quinoa or brown rice
- Guacamole or avocado slices

- Shredded spinach or lettuce.
- Grated cheese, *if desired*.
- Greek yoghurt or sour cream *(optional)*.
- Jalapenos, sliced *(optional)*.

Instructions:

Sweet Potatoes roasted:

Turn on the oven to 400 °F (200 °C).
Add the diced sweet potatoes, olive oil, chilli powder, powdered cumin, salt and pepper to a large bowl.

Sweet potatoes should be coated uniformly after tossing. On a baking sheet, arrange the sweet potatoes in a single layer.

Stirring halfway through, roast in the preheated oven for approximately 25 to 30 minutes or until they are soft but still somewhat crunchy.

Getting ready the black beans:

A little olive oil should be heated in a pan over medium heat.

Add the minced garlic and cook until fragrant for approximately 1 minute.

Black beans, ground cumin, chilli powder, salt and pepper should all be added. Stirring periodically, cook the beans for a further 5-7 minutes or until thoroughly cooked and flavorful.

Salsa preparation:

Diced tomatoes, red onion, cilantro, lime juice, salt and pepper should all be combined in a bowl. To prepare salsa, thoroughly combine.

Put together the burrito bowl:

Each dish should begin with a foundation of cooked brown rice or quinoa after which black beans and roasted sweet potatoes should be added on top.

Scoop some salsa generously on top, add grated cheese, shredded lettuce or spinach, sliced jalapenos, guacamole, avocado slices or both, as preferred.

Ready to serve your delectable Sweet Potato and Black Bean Burrito Bowl.

C. Delectable Dinners

Grilled Salmon with Fiber-Rich Veggies:
A tasty and nutritious dinner that is simple to make is grilled salmon with vegetables high in fibre. In this dish, grilled salmon is combined with a range of vibrant and healthy veggies to create a rich flavour. This is how to do it:

Ingredients:

The salmon:
- 4 salmon fillets, each weighing around 6 ounces
- Olive oil, two teaspoons
- 2 minced garlic cloves
- Lemon zest, 1 teaspoon
- Lemon juice, two teaspoons
- pepper and salt as desired

For the vegetables high in fibre:
- 200 grammes of broccoli florets
- 2 cups florets of cauliflower

- 2 cups baby carrots or carrot sticks
- 2 tablespoons of olive oil, 1 red bell pepper, 1 yellow bell Pepper, 1 zucchini and 1 yellow squash sliced
- 1/9 teaspoon dried thyme, or thyme leaves, fresh
- Pepper and salt as desired

Instructions:

400°F or 200°C or above should be the medium heat setting on your grill.

For the salmon marinade, combine the olive oil, minced garlic, lemon juice, lemon zest and salt & pepper in a small bowl.

Pour the marinade over the salmon fillets that have been placed in a shallow dish. While you prepare the vegetables, let them marinade for around 15 to 30 minutes.

Combine all the chopped vegetables for the fibre-rich veggies in a large mixing basin. Olive oil should be drizzled over the dish before adding salt, pepper and dry thyme. Toss to distribute the spice evenly over the vegetables.

To make a grill packet for the vegetables, prepare a grill basket or use aluminium foil that has holes punched in it. Put the seasoned veggies on the foil or in the grill basket.

Place the skin-side down on the grilling grate with the salmon fillets that have been marinated. Depending on the thickness of the fillets, grill the salmon for 4–5 minutes each side or until it reaches the required doneness. With a fork, it ought to flake with ease.

Cook the veggies on the grill while the salmon is cooking. For even cooking, stir them every so often. Grill the vegetables for 10 to 15 minutes, or until they are soft and slightly browned.

Salmon and vegetables should be taken off the grill.

Place the grilled salmon and the fibre-rich vegetables on a dish. If preferred, add more lemon zest or fresh herbs as a garnish. Serve and enjoy your grilled salmon dish with vegetables high in fibre!

This dish is not only tasty but also full of dietary fibre and other minerals.

Chickpea and Spinach Curry:

Here is a delicious recipe for chickpea and spinach curry.

Ingredients:

- Vegetable oil, two teaspoons
- One big onion, coarsely chopped; three cloves of minced garlic; one inch of grated ginger; one can (15 ounces); drained and washed chickpeas.
- One 14-ounce can shredded tomatoes
- One 14-ounce can coconut cream
- Curry powder, two tablespoons
- 1 teaspoon of cumin, ground
- 1 teaspoon of coriander, ground
- 12 teaspoon each of paprika and turmeric
- Cayenne pepper, 1/4 teaspoon *(modify to your taste)*.
- To taste, add salt and black pepper.
- 4 cups leafy fresh spinach
- 1/2 lemon juice
- Fresh cilantro leaves may be used as a garnish.
- Naan bread or cooked rice for serving

Instructions:

In a large skillet or pan, warm the vegetable oil over
medium heat. The chopped onion should be added and
sautéed for approximately 5 minutes or until transparent.

Add the grated ginger and garlic powder, stir and simmer
for an additional one to two minutes or until fragrant.

Add the cayenne pepper, salt, black pepper, turmeric,
paprika, curry powder, powdered cumin and ground
coriander. To uniformly coat the onions and spices, stir
thoroughly. To toast the spices, cook for 2 to 3 minutes.

Add the tomato juice and diced tomatoes. Stir to
incorporate the spice blend.

Stir the chickpeas into the tomato-spice mixture after
adding them to the pan.

Add the coconut milk, then gently boil the mixture.
Stirring regularly, let it boil for 10 to 15 minutes or until the
sauce thickens and the chickpeas are well heated.

Fresh spinach leaves should be added to the pan and cooked for a further two to three minutes or until they wilt and soften.

Stir the curry after adding the juice of half a lemon to bring out the flavour of the fresh citrus.

After tasting the curry, add more salt, pepper or spices if necessary to improve the flavour.

With warm rice or naan bread, serve the chickpea and spinach curry. If desired, garnish with fresh cilantro leaves.

Lemon Herb Chicken with Asparagus:
A tasty and nutritious meal like Lemon Herb Chicken with Asparagus is ideal for a fast evening meal. Here is a simple recipe you might try:

Ingredients:

The chicken with lemon and herbs is:
- 4 skinless, boneless breasts of chicken
- Olive oil, two teaspoons
- 2 minced garlic cloves

- 1 lemon, juiced and zested
- Oregano, dry, 1 teaspoon
- One tablespoon of dried thyme
- Pepper and salt as desired

Regarding the asparagus:
- 1 bunch of trimmed fresh asparagus
- Olive oil, two teaspoons
- pepper and salt as desired
- Sliced thinly for garnish, one lemon

Instructions:

Preheat the oven to 375 degrees Fahrenheit (190 degrees Celsius).

Chicken preparation: Olive oil, minced garlic, lemon juice, zest, dried thyme, salt and pepper should all be combined in a small bowl.

Chicken breasts should be placed in a shallow dish or a zip-top bag and covered with the lemon-herb marinade. For at least 30 minutes, marinate the dish in the refrigerator with the bag closed or covered.

The flavour will be improved if you marinate the food for many hours or overnight.

Asparagus preparation: On a baking sheet, mix the trimmed asparagus with olive oil, salt and pepper while the chicken is marinating. They should be dispersed in one layer.

Asparagus and Chicken are cooked together on the same baking sheet once the chicken has been taken out of the marinade. Use a second baking sheet for the chicken if yours is already crowded. Any leftover marinade should be drizzled over the chicken and asparagus.

Bake: Bake the chicken in the preheated oven for 25 to 30 minutes or until it is well cooked *(the internal temperature reaches 165°F or 74°C)* and the asparagus is crisp-tender.

Remove the chicken and asparagus from the oven to serve as a garnish. If preferred, garnish with lemon slices and extra herbs.

To serve, arrange the chicken and asparagus on a plate and top with any pan juices. Serve warm with your preferred side dishes, such rice or a simple salad.

Take pleasure in your flavorful and wholesome Lemon Herb Chicken with Asparagus! This recipe is a fantastic option for a healthy supper since it is tasty, low in carbohydrates and rich in protein.

Chapter 4: Probiotic Power

A. Fermented Favourites

Homemade Kimchi:

A tasty and wholesome Korean side dish called homemade kimchi is created from fermented vegetables, usually Korean radishes and Napa cabbage. Here is a simple kimchi recipe that you may use at home. Remember that there are several regional and individual versions of this traditional cuisine; this is only one example.

Ingredients:

- 1 medium-sized *(approximately 2 pounds)* Napa cabbage
- 1/fourth cup kosher salt
- Water to be soaked in.
- 1 Korean radish or daikon radish
- 4 to 5 onions
- One little carrot, *optional*
- 5-7 minced garlic cloves
- 1 chopped, thumb-sized piece of ginger
- 3–4 teaspoons of gochugaru, a Korean red pepper flakes

- For a non-vegetarian variation, add Two teaspoons of fish sauce.
- Sugar, 1 to 2 teaspoons
- Soy sauce, 1-2 teaspoons *(optional)*
- *(Optional)* 1-2 teaspoons of seafood brine for added umami flavour
- For blending the spice paste, use 1 cup of water.

Instructions:

Get the cabbage ready:

Napa cabbage should be chopped into bite-sized pieces after being cut in half lengthwise.

Put water in a big dish and dissolve 1/4 cup of kosher salt in it. To achieve equal salting, flip the cabbage pieces regularly while soaking them in the salty water for one to two hours. Drain after giving the cabbage a good rinse.

Get the vegetables ready:

The daikon radish should be peeled and chopped into thin matchsticks.
Scallions should be cut into 2-inch chunks.

Peel and chop a carrot into thin matchsticks if you're using one.

Creating the seasoning paste:

Minced garlic, ginger, sugar, Korean red pepper flakes, soy sauce, fish sauce and seafood brine may all be combined in a blender or food processor. When you have a smooth paste, add roughly 1 cup of water and mix again.

Combine all the ingredients:

Combine the drained cabbage, daikon radish, scallions and carrot (*if using*) in a large mixing bowl.

Put on gloves and rub the spice paste into the veggies until they are well covered. Because the red pepper flakes might be hot, avoid touching your face or eyes while doing this.

Place in Jar:

In an airtight container or clean glass jar, pack the kimchi mixture firmly. As the kimchi ferments, it will grow, so leave some room at the top.

Fermentation:

To start the fermentation process, let the jar at room temperature for one to two days. After that, keep it in the fridge for 3–7 days—or even longer—to give it time to continue fermenting. It will get tangier and more delicious as it ferments for a longer period of time.

Enjoy: You may now enjoy your handmade kimchi! You may use it on top of rice, in stir-fries, soups or as a side dish.

During fermentation, don't forget to burp the jar periodically by opening it to let any trapped gas out. As a result, the jar is less likely to rupture from the gases created during fermentation.

Kombucha Brewing Guide:

A fermented tea beverage known as kombucha has grown in popularity due to its intriguing flavour and possible health advantages. Here is a simple recipe from a kombucha brewing guide to get you going. Please be aware that this recipe requires you already own or have access to a kombucha SCOBY *(Symbiotic Culture Of Bacteria and Yeast)*.

Ingredients:

To start the fermentation:

- 2 teaspoons of loose tea or 4-6 black or green tea bags
- 1 cup of sugar, granulated
- SYMBIOTIC CULTURE OF BACTERIA AND YEAST (SCOBY) One.
- 2 cups of starter tea *(raw kombucha from the store or previously brewed kombucha)*.
- Glass or ceramic 1-gallon container Cloth or paper towel and a rubber band for covering the container.
- Purified water

For the optional second fermentation:

- Fruit, herbs, spices and other flavours
- Reversible glass bottles

Instructions:

Initially Fermenting:

To avoid contamination, start by carefully cleaning all of the equipment. Tea bags *(or loose tea)* should be steeped in 4-6 cups of boiling water for 5-7 minutes.

Until the sugar is totally dissolved, add it and stir. The SCOBY will be fed by this.

Wait until the tea is at room temperature. The SCOBY may be harmed by adding hot tea to it.

Transfer the tea to the gallon glass jar after it has cooled.

Fill the jar with the beginning tea and SCOBY. Normally, the SCOBY will float on top.

Fill the jar up to the top with distilled water, leaving approximately an inch of space.

With a rubber band, cover the jar with a cloth or paper towel. This keeps dirt and other particles out while allowing the kombucha to breathe.

For fermentation, put the jar in a warm, dark location (70–75°F; 21–24°C). According to your taste, let it ferment for 7 to 14 days. It will be less sweet the longer it ferments.

Taste your kombucha after the fermenting period has passed as desired. It's time to go to the second fermentation if you find it to be satisfactory. If not, you may give it more time to ferment.

Optional second fermentation:

Take the SCOBY out of the first fermentation jar along with around 2 cups of the liquid. To use as a starting for your subsequent batch, set them aside.

Fill the kombucha bottles with the flavourings of your choice. Fruits, herbs, spices and fruit juices may all be considered here. Try out several flavour combinations to discover your favourites.

The fermented kombucha should be poured into the bottles, allowing approximately an inch of room at the top.

With the flip-top lids, securely cap the bottles.

Depending on the desired amount of carbonation, let the second fermentation last 2 to 7 days at room temperature. Keep the bottles out of the sun's direct rays.

After the second fermentation, chill the kombucha in the refrigerator to slow the fermentation and prepare it for serving.

Pour the kombucha into a glass and discard any debris that collects at the bottom of the container upon serving.

Enjoy the kombucha you brewed at home! Do note that it could take a few batches to get the flavour and fizziness just right for you. To avoid infection, handle the SCOBY with clean hands and utensils at all times.

Greek Tzatziki Sauce:

Delicious Greek tzatziki sauce is produced with yoghurt, cucumber, garlic and spices. It is often served as a dip, a topping for gyros and souvlaki or with grilled meats. An easy recipe for homemade tzatziki sauce is provided below:

Ingredients:

- 1 peeled and grated cucumber
- Greek yoghurt in two cups
- 2 minced garlic cloves
- Extra virgin olive oil, 1 tablespoon

- 1 tablespoon of lemon juice, fresh
- 1 teaspoon dried dill or 1 tablespoon minced fresh dill
- 1 tablespoon finely chopped fresh mint
- pepper and salt as desired

Instructions:

Grate the cucumber first. You may use a food processor with a grating attachment or a box grater. After being grated, lay the cucumber over a bowl in a fine-mesh sieve or cheesecloth to drain any extra juice. By doing this, you can keep your tzatziki from being overly watery.

Greek yoghurt, minced garlic, olive oil and lemon juice should all be mixed together in a bowl. Blend well.

Use your palms or the back of a spoon to push the grated cucumber to remove any liquid that is still there. To the yoghurt mixture, include the drained cucumber.

Add the mint and fresh dill, if using. The traditional herb for tzatziki is dill, but mint gives it a cool edge. To taste, add salt and pepper to the food. Do not immediately oversalt the sauce since it will gain flavour as it rests.

All of the ingredients should be well mixed. Taste the tzatziki and, *if required*, add additional lemon juice, garlic or herbs to change the flavour.

To enable the flavours to merge, cover the bowl with plastic wrap or a lid and place it in the refrigerator for at least an hour. If you can put it in the fridge for a few hours or overnight, the better.

Give the tzatziki one more swirl before serving and add a little olive oil to the top for a great finishing touch.

Tzatziki is excellent as a sauce for grilled meats, a dip for pita bread or veggies or a topping for sandwiches and wraps.

B. Gut-Boosting Soups

Creamy Butternut Squash Soup:

A delightful and cosy recipe, particularly in the autumn and winter, is creamy butternut squash soup. See simple recipe for this filling soup:

Ingredients:

- 1 medium butternut squash, weighing about 2 pounds.
- Olive oil, two teaspoons
- 1 chopped medium onion
- 2 minced garlic cloves
- 1 peeled and sliced carrot
- 1 sliced celery stalk
- 1 apple, cored, peeled and diced *(for sweetness, optional)*.
- 4 cups of chicken or veggie broth
- One tablespoon of dried thyme
- 1/8 teaspoon cinnamon powder
- 1/4 teaspoon of nutmeg, ground
- Pepper and salt as desired
- 1 cup heavy cream *(or a vegan substitute that doesn't contain dairy)*.
- Croutons or toasted pumpkin seeds as a garnish *(optional)*

Instructions:

Set your oven's temperature to 375°F (190°C). Scoop off the seeds and pulp from the butternut squash after cutting it in half lengthwise. If you'd like, you may save the seeds for toasting later.

On a baking sheet, spread the squash halves, drizzle with 1 tablespoon of olive oil and season with salt and pepper. 45 minutes should be allotted for roasting or until the meat is soft and readily punctured with a fork.

The remaining 1 tablespoon of olive oil should be heated over medium heat in a big saucepan or Dutch oven while the squash is roasting.

Add the chopped carrot, celery, apple, onion and garlic, and sauté for approximately 5-7 minutes or until the veggies are softened.

Scoop out the flesh of the butternut squash once it has finished roasting, then add it to the saucepan with the sautéed veggies after it has cooled somewhat. Throw away the skin.

Add the dried thyme, ground cinnamon and grated nutmeg to the vegetable or chicken stock before pouring it in. Stir well.

Once it begins to boil, turn the heat down to low, cover the pot, and let the mixture simmer for 20 to 25 minutes or until the veggies are all very soft.

Carefully purée the soup in an immersion blender until it is smooth and creamy. Alternately, you might add the soup in stages to a blender, puree it and then add the blended soup back to the saucepan.

The heavy cream *(or dairy-free substitute)* should be stirred in after the soup has been heated gradually until it is hot but not boiling.
To taste, add salt and pepper to the food.

If preferred, top the hot, creamy butternut squash soup with toasted pumpkin seeds or croutons.
Take pleasure in your homemade butternut squash soup! It works well as a beginning or a hearty supper by itself.

Probiotic Tomato Basil Bisque:

Probiotic Tomato Basil Bisque is a delectable and nutritious soup that mixes the flavours of fresh basil and ripe tomatoes with the benefits of probiotics for the digestive system. Here is a dish you should try:

Ingredients:

- Olive oil, two teaspoons
- 1 chopped medium onion
- 2 minced garlic cloves
- Diced tomatoes in two *(14.5-ounce)* cans, ideally fire-roasted
- 6 ounces of tomato paste in one can
- 4 cups of veggie broth
- 1 cup of dairy-free or plain Greek yoghurt for vegans
- chopped half a cup of fresh basil leaves
- Oregano, dry, 1 teaspoon
- Pepper and salt as desired
- Yoghurt or kefir with probiotics as a garnish *(optional)*
- Basil leaves for garnish, fresh
- For serving, croutons or toasted bread *are optional*.

Instructions:

Olive oil should be heated in a large saucepan over medium heat. Cook for approximately 5 minutes after adding the chopped onion or until it becomes translucent.

When aromatic, add the minced garlic to the saucepan and cook for an additional one to two minutes.

Add the tomato paste and chopped tomatoes with their juices. 5 minutes of cooking will enable the flavours to mingle.

Salt, pepper, dried oregano and vegetable broth should all be added. After bringing the mixture to a boil, lower the heat, cover the pan and simmer the mixture for 15 to 20 minutes, stirring now and again.

Carefully purée the soup using an immersion blender until it is smooth. As an alternative, you may add the soup in stages to a blender, but you should use caution since hot liquids might spatter.

Return the smoothed-out soup to the pot and heat it gently.

Greek yoghurt and fresh basil leaves are then combined. Allow the soup to heat through and the flavours to meld for an extra five minutes of cooking.

If necessary, add more salt and pepper to the dish's flavouring.

Pour bowls with the probiotic tomato basil bisque. If preferred, add a dollop of probiotic-rich yoghurt or kefir, a sprig of fresh basil and some croutons or toasted bread to each dish for texture.

Your probiotic-rich tomato basil bisque should be served hot.

To be tasty, this soup also has probiotics from the yoghurt, which helps improve intestinal health. Feel free to modify the seasoning or add more herbs and spices to the dish to suit your preferences.

Miso Noodle Soup:
A wonderful and calming Japanese cuisine that is simple to prepare at home is miso noodle soup. Noodles and a variety of toppings are generally included, along with a flavorful broth prepared with miso paste. Here is a simple miso noodle soup recipe:

Ingredients:

To the broth:

- 4 cups of chicken or veggie broth
- Miso paste, either red or white depending on your desire, 3 teaspoons.
- 2 minced garlic cloves
- 1 tablespoon freshly grated ginger
- Soy sauce, two teaspoons
- Sesame oil, 1 tablespoon

For the toppings and noodles:

- 8 ounces of your favourite dry noodle, such as soba or udon
- 1 cup of sliced mushrooms, preferably shiitake or cremini
- 1 cup of chopped spinach or bok choy
- 1/2 cup of green onions, thinly sliced
- Cooked chicken or tofu cubes *(optional for additional protein)*.
- Seaweed nori sheets for garnish
- Sesame seeds for decoration

Instructions:

Get the noodles ready:

Noodles should be cooked as directed on the box until they are al dente.
To stop the cooking, drain the noodles and rinse them in cool water. Put them apart.

Get the broth ready:

Sesame oil should be heated in a medium-sized saucepan over medium heat.

Embrace grated ginger and chopped garlic. Sauté until aromatic for around 1-2 minutes.

Add the broth, then gently boil the mixture.

Dissolve Miso Paste

A few tablespoons of the hot broth from the saucepan should be whisked into the miso paste in a small bowl until everything is thoroughly mixed and smooth.

Re-add the miso paste that has been dissolved, then blend everything together.

Include toppings and soy sauce:

To enable the flavours to blend, add the soy sauce to the broth and let it boil for around 5 minutes.
The broth should now include the chopped mushrooms and bok choy *(or spinach)*. Allow them to simmer for 3 to 5 minutes or until they are cooked.

Build the soup:

Put the cooked noodles into dishes for dishing.
Over the noodles, pour the heated broth containing the mushrooms and greens.

Add chicken or tofu (optional): Add cooked chicken or tofu cubes to the soup bowls if using.

Serve and Garnish: Top each dish with sesame seeds, chopped green onions and broken nori sheets.
Enjoy your hot miso noodle soup after serving!

Chapter 5: Healing Herbs and Spices

A. Flavorful Infusions

Turmeric and Ginger Tea:

A calming and tasty beverage with possible health advantages, turmeric and ginger tea. Both ginger and turmeric are thought to have antioxidant and anti-inflammatory qualities. A simple recipe for this tea:

Ingredients:

- 1-2 inches of freshly peeled and sliced ginger root *(adjust to taste)*.
- Use 1/2 to 1 teaspoon of powdered turmeric instead of the raw, peeled and grated turmeric root.
- 2 to 3 cups of water
- 1 to 2 tablespoons of optionally sweetened honey or maple syrup
- Lemon juice that has just been squeezed *(optional; for flavour)*.
- A dash of black pepper, *which is optional* but helps the body absorb turmeric's curcumin.

Instructions:

Boil some water first. On the stove, you may use a kettle or a saucepan.

Prepare the ginger and turmeric while the water is heating. If using fresh roots, grate the turmeric and cut the ginger into slices. Skip this step if you're using ground turmeric.

Add the grated turmeric and ginger slices to the boiling water after it has reached a rolling boil. For approximately 10-15 minutes, turn the heat down to low, cover the pot and let the mixture simmer.

The flavours will be able to permeate the water as a result.

After the tea has simmered, drain it to get rid of the chunks of ginger and turmeric. You may use a tea infuser or a fine-mesh strainer.

While the tea is still warm, add honey or maple syrup if you want to sweeten it. Your preferred level of sweetness should be used.

Add a sprinkle of black pepper to the tea to improve the absorption of curcumin, the key ingredient in turmeric. Black pepper includes piperine, which may increase curcumin's absorption.

To add flavour and vitamin C to your cup of turmeric and ginger tea, you may optionally pour some fresh lemon juice into it.

Enjoy the soothing and maybe healthy benefits of your hot cup of turmeric and ginger tea.

Remember that the quantity of ginger and turmeric you use and your personal tastes might affect how strong the tea is. You can experiment with various flavour ingredients like cinnamon or cloves for added warmth and flavour by adjusting the proportions to your taste.

Rosemary Roasted Vegetables:
A tasty and nutritious side dish that goes well with a variety of main dishes is rosemary roasted veggies. Here is a simple method for roasting veggies with rosemary:

Ingredients:

- Veggies of several varieties *(including potatoes, carrots, bell peppers, zucchini and onions)*
- Olive oil, 2 to 3 teaspoons
- Minced garlic from 2 to 3 cloves *(optional)*.
- 1 teaspoon dried rosemary or 1-2 teaspoons chopped fresh rosemary.
- Pepper and salt as desired

Instructions:

Turn on the oven to 425 °F (220 °C).

Your veggies should be washed, peeled *(if required)* and chopped into uniform-sized pieces. You may combine a few of your preferred veggies. Potatoes, carrots, bell peppers, zucchini and onions are a few of the often used ingredients.

Olive oil, minced garlic *(if used)*, chopped rosemary, salt and pepper should all be combined with the chopped veggies in a large mixing dish. Combine everything and stir until the oil and spices are evenly distributed among the veggies.

On a baking sheet, arrange the seasoned veggies in a single layer. To keep things from sticking, line the baking sheet with parchment paper or gently oil it.

Roast the veggies for 25 to 35 minutes or until they are soft and have a lovely golden brown colour, on a baking sheet in a preheated oven.

To achieve consistent cooking, toss or turn the veggies with a spatula a couple of times during roasting.

Remove the veggies from the oven after they have been roasted to the desired degree of doneness.

If necessary, add more salt and pepper after tasting the food.

Place the rosemary-roasted veggies on a serving dish and, *if preferred*, top with more fresh rosemary.

Serve this meal hot as a side dish to your preferred main entrée. These roasted veggies go well with grilled steak, roasted chicken, or even just by themselves.

Cilantro Lime Quinoa:

Cilantro Lime Quinoa is a tasty and nourishing side dish that goes well with a variety of entrees, particularly those with a Mexican or Southwestern theme. You might try the following easy recipe:

Ingredients:

- Quinoa in a cup
- 2 cups of vegetable or water broth
- Chopped half a cup of fresh cilantro
- Juice from one or two limes, to taste
- Zest from one lime
- Minced garlic from 2 cloves
- 1 teaspoon of olive oil
- To taste with salt and pepper

Alternative toppings:

- Tomato slices
- Green onions, cut up
- Chopped avocado
- Jalapenos in slices
- Shredded cheese
- Greek yoghurt or sour cream

Instructions:

Quinoa should be rinsed in cold water to get rid of any bitterness before cooking. It should be thoroughly drained.

Quinoa is prepared by placing rinsed quinoa, water or vegetable broth and stirring to incorporate. Over a medium-high flame, bring it to a boil. For approximately 15-20 minutes or until the quinoa has absorbed all the liquid and is soft, reduce the heat to low, cover the pan and simmer.

Quinoa should be fluffed after being cooked. After being taken off the heat, quinoa should be left covered for five minutes. To separate the grains, fluff it with a fork after that.

The cilantro-lime dressing: Lime juice, lime zest, garlic, olive oil, salt and pepper should all be combined in a small bowl.

Fluffed and cooked quinoa should be added to a large mixing dish along with the dressing.

While the quinoa is still warm, drizzle the dressing with the cilantro and lime. As you blend, make sure the dressing is spread evenly.

Cilantro, chopped: Gently incorporate the quinoa mixture with the chopped cilantro. The flavours will be infused since the quinoa's heat will cause the cilantro to somewhat wilt.

Serve: You can either serve the cilantro-lime quinoa warm or at room temperature. Toppings like diced tomatoes, chopped green onions, sliced avocado, sliced jalapenos, grated cheese or a dollop of sour cream or Greek yoghurt may be added as desired.

You can use the cilantro-lime quinoa as a side dish for your favourite main dishes, such grilled chicken or fish or as a foundation for burrito bowls. It may also be eaten as a stand-alone dish and is perfect for meal preparation.

B. Herbal Remedies

Peppermint Soothing Smoothie:

When it's hot outside or you're feeling queasy, a peppermint calming smoothie may be a cold, comforting beverage. Simple recipe you might try:

Ingredients:

- 1 cup of plain Greek yoghurt *(or a vegan dairy-free substitute)*.
- 1/2 cup of milk, either dairy or vegan
- One ripe banana
- Add peppermint essence to taste, about half a teaspoon.
- 1 tablespoon of maple syrup or honey, tasted,
- Ice cubes, 1/2 cup
- A few fresh mint leaves, optionally, for garnish and added freshness.
- Vanilla extract, 1/4 teaspoon *(optional)*

Instructions:

Start by putting the milk, ripe banana, peppermint extract, honey or maple syrup, Greek yoghurt *(or a substitute)* and ice cubes in a blender.

You may also add a little bit of vanilla essence for flavour if you'd like.

Until the mixture is smooth and creamy, blend all the ingredients on high speed. If you want to be sure that everything is well combined, you may need to pause and scrape the sides of the blender.

To your pleasure, taste the smoothie and adjust the sweetness and peppermint flavour. If needed, increase the amount of honey or peppermint essence.

Pour the smoothie into a glass as soon as you're pleased with the flavour and consistency.
You may add some fresh mint leaves as a garnish to the smoothie if you have some on hand.

Serve your Peppermint Soothing Smoothie right away!

Thanks to the peppermint, this smoothie has a calming effect in addition to being tasty. It's excellent for settling an upset stomach or just as a cool treat.

Chamomile and Lavender Sleep Elixir:

A lovely method to encourage relaxation and improve the quality of your sleep is to make a chamomile and lavender sleep elixir. The relaxing and soothing qualities of chamomile and lavender are well recognised. The following is a straightforward recipe for a chamomile and lavender sleep elixir:

Ingredients:

- Water, 1 cup
- Two teaspoons of chamomile flowers, dried
- 1 tablespoon of lavender buds, dried
- 1-2 tablespoons of optionally sweetened honey
- A little pot
- A strainer with fine mesh
- A storage container made of heat-resistant glass

Instructions:

Water to Boil: In a small saucepan, bring one cup of water to a boil.

Add herbs: As soon as the water reaches a rolling boil, take it from the heat and stir in the dried chamomile flowers and lavender buds.

Steep: Place a cover on the pan and allow the herbs to steep in the boiling water for 10 to 15 minutes. This enables the flavours and healthy ingredients to permeate the water.

After steeping, pour the liquid into a heatproof glass jar or container using a fine-mesh strainer. In order to extract all of the infused liquid, be sure to push firmly on the herbs. Throw out the used herbs.

Sweeten *(Optional)*: While the infused liquid is still warm, add 1-2 tablespoons of honey if you want a little sweeter elixir. The honey must be thoroughly dissolved by stirring.

Elixir should be allowed to cool to room temperature.

Storage: You may keep the elixir in the refrigerator for up to a week once it has cooled. Make careful to properly cap the jar or container.

Usage:

About 30 to 60 minutes before bedtime, sip a small cup *(about 1/4 to 1/2 cup)* of this chamomile and lavender sleep elixir.

If you want it hot, you may rewarm it before drinking it.

To get the most calming benefits from your elixir, remember to rest and unwind while drinking it.

Although chamomile and lavender are widely acknowledged to be safe for the majority of individuals, it is advisable to speak with a healthcare provider before incorporating herbal treatments into your regimen if you have allergies or are on drugs.

Basil and Garlic Gut-Healing Pesto:

If you add gut-friendly ingredients, basil and garlic pesto may be a delectable and healthy complement to your meals. It also has some gut-healing characteristics. Here is a recipe for a pesto that can help your digestive system:

Ingredients:

- 2 cups of basil leaves, fresh
- 3–4 garlic cloves
- Extra virgin olive oil, half a cup
- Uncooked pine nuts or walnuts, half a cup
- If you're lactose intolerant, eliminate *the optional* 1/4 cup of grated Parmesan cheese.

- Lemon juice from one
- 1/4 teaspoon black pepper, 1/2 teaspoon sea salt and 1 teaspoon lemon zest.
- 1 tablespoon maple syrup or honey *(optional, for extra sweetness)*
- 1 teaspoon ground flaxseed *(for fibre addition)*
- Chia seeds, 1 tablespoon *(for more fibre and omega-3 fatty acids)*

Instructions:

The nuts may be toasted in a dry pan over medium heat for a few minutes or until they start to become gently brown. Although it's optional, this step might improve the pesto's flavour.

Wash the basil leaves and blot them dry with a paper towel to prepare the basil.

Blend Basil leaves, garlic cloves, roasted almonds, lemon juice, lemon zest, salt, pepper and optional honey or maple syrup should all be combined in a food processor or blender. Pulse the mixture until it begins to disintegrate.

Olive Oil: Slowly drizzle in the extra-virgin olive oil while the food processor or blender is running to get the appropriate consistency for the pesto. In order to make sure everything is well blended, you may need to pause and scrape down the container's edges.

Add ground flaxseed and chia seeds after the pesto has been well mixed and is smooth. These components are rich in omega-3 fatty acids and fibre, both of which are good for gut health. To mix them into the pesto, blend them quickly once more.

Adapt the seasoning by tasting the pesto and adding more salt, pepper or sweetness as desired. For added flavour, you may also add additional lemon zest or juice.

Cheese, *optional*: At this point, if you're using Parmesan cheese, add it to the food processor and pulse until everything is well blended. You may leave out the cheese if you're vegan or avoid dairy.

Dispatch or Hold: Put the pesto in a refrigerator-safe container after transferring it there. It is available right away for use as a spaghetti sauce, sandwich spread, topping for grilled veggies and fresh bread dip. In the refrigerator, it will last for about a week.

Chapter 6: Desserts with Benefits

A. Sweet Treats

Blueberry Almond Chia Pudding:

Chia pudding with blueberries and almonds is a tasty and healthy alternative for breakfast or a snack. For a fast and practical supper, it is simple to prepare the night before. I've got a quick recipe for you:

Ingredients:

- Chia seeds, 1/4 cup
- 1 cup of your choice of milk, such as almond milk
- One-half teaspoon of vanilla extract
- 1 tablespoon maple syrup or honey (modify to taste)
- 1/2 cup blueberries, either fresh or frozen
- Almond slices *(for decoration)*
- Fresh blueberries *(optional garnish)*

Instructions:

Chia seeds, almond milk, vanilla extract, honey and maple syrup should all be combined in a mixing dish. To make sure the chia seeds are dispersed equally, stir well.

After letting the mixture settle for 5 to 10 minutes, stir it once more. The chia seeds won't bunch up as a result of this.

Refrigerate the bowl for at least two hours or overnight, covered with plastic wrap or a lid. The chia seeds will absorb the liquid during this time and thicken to produce a pudding-like consistency.

Take the chia pudding out of the fridge and give it a nice stir just before serving.

Layer the blueberries and chia pudding in serving glasses or bowls. The bottom of the glass may be filled with blueberries, followed by a layer of chia pudding and additional blueberries. Continue as necessary.

Sliced almonds and fresh blueberries may be sprinkled on top of the custard for flavour and texture.

Chia pudding with blueberries and almonds may be kept in the fridge for up to three to four days before serving. When serving leftovers, you may need to add a little additional almond milk since the longer it sits, the thicker it will get.

Chocolate Avocado Mousse:

Chocolate avocado mousse is a simple, delicious and healthful dessert. It's ideal for anyone seeking a mousse substitute that is dairy-free, vegan or low in sugar. I've got a quick recipe for you:

Ingredients:

- Two mature avocados.
- Unsweetened cocoa powder, 1/4 cup
- 1/4 cup agave nectar or maple syrup *(modify to taste)*.
- Any non-dairy milk, or 1/4 cup of almond milk.
- Vanilla extract, 1 teaspoon
- Add a little salt
- Berry, chopped almonds, shredded coconut or whipped coconut cream are optional toppings.

Instructions:

Remove the pits from the avocados by cutting them in half, then scoop the flesh into a food processor or blender.

The avocados should also be mixed with cocoa powder, maple syrup *(or agave nectar)*, almond milk, vanilla essence and a dash of salt.

Until the mixture is smooth and creamy, combine all the ingredients in a blender. To make sure everything is well blended, you may need to pause and scrape down the sides of the blender or food processor.

If required, add additional maple syrup or cocoa powder after tasting the mousse to your desired level of sweetness or chocolate flavour.

Transfer the mousse to serving plates or small bowls after it is flavorful and smooth.

Before serving, place the mousse in the refrigerator for at least 30 minutes. This aids in its firming and cooling.

You may top the dish with your preferred ingredients just before serving, such as fresh fruit, chopped almonds, shredded coconut or a dollop of coconut cream.

Enjoy your mousse of chocolate and avocado! It tastes finest when cold.

You can be inventive with this recipe since it is so adaptable. You may also play around with other garnish and adaptations, such as adding a dash of espresso powder or a touch of cinnamon for flavour.

Berry Sorbet:

Ingredients:

2 cups of mixed berries, which may include any mixture of strawberries, blueberries, raspberries and blackberries.
0.5 cups of granulated sugar, taste-tested
0.5 cups of water
1 tablespoon of optional fresh lemon juice
1 teaspoon optional vanilla extract

Instructions:

To prepare the berries, properly wash them in a washbasin with cold running water. Eliminate any leaves or stalks.

For this dish, berries may be either fresh or frozen.

Create a simple syrup by mixing water and granulated sugar in a small pot. Stirring constantly, heat over medium heat until the sugar is fully dissolved. Take it off the stove and let it cool to room temperature. You need this simple syrup.

Blend the Berries: Use a food processor or blender to combine the berries. You may save a few berries for later garnish if you'd like. The berries should be mixed with the lemon juice and vanilla essence *(if using)*.

Pour the cooled simple syrup into the blender along with the berries to add simple syrup. Blend the ingredients until they are well-combined and smooth.

Taste the mixture and, if necessary, add additional sugar or lemon juice to change the sweetness or sharpness.

Optional straining: Pour the mixture through a fine-mesh strainer or cheesecloth into a clean basin for a smoother sorbet free of berry particles. Remove any seeds or particles by pressing the mixture through with a spoon or spatula.

Refrigerate the mixture for at least two hours or until it is well cold, with the bowl covered with plastic wrap.

Freeze: After the liquid has cooled, pour it into an ice cream machine and churn it as directed by the manufacturer. Normally, this takes 20 to 25 minutes.

To serve, move the sorbet that has been churned to an airtight container and freeze it for a further 2-4 hours or until it is solid.

When it's time to serve, ladle the berry sorbet into bowls or cones. Garnish as desired. If desired, add some fresh berries as a garnish.

B. Gut-Friendly Baking

Gluten-Free Banana Bread:

It's ideal for anybody searching for a great banana bread substitute or for those with gluten concerns.

Ingredients:

- 3 mashed, ripe bananas
- Two huge eggs
- Melted coconut oil or vegetable oil, 1/3 cup
- 1/2 cup maple syrup or honey
- Vanilla extract, 1 teaspoon
- 1 1/2 cups all-purpose gluten-free flour *(if it doesn't already include xanthan gum, add 1/2 teaspoon)*;
- One tablespoon of baking soda

- 14 teaspoon salt and 12 teaspoon optional ground cinnamon
- 0.5 cup chopped nuts, such as walnuts or pecans or *(optional)* Chocolate chips.

Instructions:

Turn on the oven to 350 °F (175 °C). For easy removal, grease or line a 4x8-inch loaf pan with parchment paper.

Use a fork to mash the ripe bananas in a mixing dish until they are mostly smooth.

The mashed bananas should be combined with the eggs, heated coconut oil *(or vegetable oil)*, honey *(or maple syrup)* and vanilla essence. All wet elements should be well mixed after mixing.

Mix the gluten-free flour, baking soda, salt and ground cinnamon *(if using)* in a separate basin.

When the batter is well blended, gradually add the dry components to the wet ones while stirring. Be cautious not to overmix; just combine the ingredients enough to combine them.

Fold any nuts or chocolate chips you're using now into the batter. Spread the batter evenly as you pour it into the prepared loaf pan.

A toothpick or cake tester put into the centre of the bread should come out clean and without any wet batter (*moist crumbs are OK*). This should take between 55 and 65 minutes in a preheated oven.

When ready, take the banana bread out of the oven and let it cool for approximately 10 minutes in the pan. After that, move it to a wire rack to finish cooling.

Slice and serve after it has cooled. Enjoy your banana bread without gluten!

This banana bread recipe is not only tasty but also adaptable. By using your own mix-ins, such as chocolate chips, chopped almonds or dried fruits, you can make it your own. It's ideal as a dessert, a snack or for breakfast.

Probiotic Yogurt Parfait Cheesecake:

The creamy deliciousness of cheesecake is combined with the health advantages of yoghurt and probiotics to create a probiotic yoghurt parfait cheesecake. Here is a recipe for a sweet that is both tasty and healthy:

Ingredients:

Within the Crust:

Graham cracker crumbs, One and 1/2 cups

14 cup of melted butter

Two teaspoons of sugar

When making the cheesecake filling:

16 oz *(2 cups)* softened cream cheese

Plain Greek yoghurt, either full-fat or low-fat, one cup

50 g of sugar

Two huge eggs

Vanilla extract, 1 teaspoon

2 tablespoons of regular flour

1/2 cup yoghurt with active cultures or kefir that is high in probiotics

Topping for the yoghurt parfait:

- 1 1/2 cups yoghurt with active cultures or kefir that is high in probiotics
- Strawberries, blueberries, raspberries and other fresh fruit
- For drizzling, use honey or maple syrup
- *(Optional)* Granola for crunchier flavour

Instructions:

Get the oven ready: Set your oven's temperature to 325 °F (160 °C).

Get the crust ready: The sugar, melted butter and graham cracker crumbs should be combined in a mixing basin. Mix just enough to coat the crumbs all over.

To create the crust, press the mixture firmly into the bottom of a 9-inch (23 cm) springform pan.

The crust has to bake for approximately 10 minutes to solidify. While you make the filling, take it out of the oven and let it cool.

Make the cheesecake filling:

Cream the softened cream cheese in a large mixing bowl
until it is smooth and creamy.

Add the sugar, eggs, vanilla extract, flour and plain Greek
yoghurt. Mix everything together well until the mixture is
smooth.
Add the yoghurt that is high in probiotics and gently mix it
in.

Put Together and Bake:

Over the chilled graham cracker crust in the springform
pan, pour the cheesecake filling.

To get rid of any air bubbles, tap the pan on the counter.
When the sides are set but the centre still jiggles slightly,
bake in the preheated oven for 45 to 50 minutes.

After turning off the oven, leave the door ajar and the
cheesecake inside to gently cool for approximately an hour.

When the cheesecake is completely cold and set, remove it from the oven and chill it for at least 4 hours or overnight.

Make the Yoghurt Parfait Topping:

Spread a layer of probiotic-rich yoghurt *(kefir or yoghurt with active cultures)* on top of the cheesecake after it is cooled and prepared to be served.

Add your preferred fresh berries to the yoghurt as decoration. Add some honey or maple syrup for additional richness.

Granola may be *optionally* added for crunch and texture.

Serve: Slice and serve your probiotic yoghurt parfait cheesecake and enjoy the amazing flavour combinations and advantages to your health.

This cheesecake, which blends the richness of cheesecake with the probiotic benefits of yoghurt and the freshness of berries, is a delicious treat. It's not only tasty; it's also healthy.

Spiced Carrot and Walnut Muffins:

Ingredients:

Those muffins:
- 2 cups of general-purpose flour
- Baking powder, 1 1/2 tablespoons
- A half-teaspoon of baking soda
- 1 teaspoon ground cinnamon and half a teaspoon of salt
- 1/8 teaspoon of nutmeg, ground
- 1/8 teaspoon of ginger powder
- 1/4 teaspoon of cloves, ground
- 12 cups softened unsalted butter
- 1 cup sugar, granulated
- Two huge eggs
- Vanilla extract, 1 teaspoon
- 1-2 medium carrots, in 1 1/2 cups of shredded carrots
- Chopped walnuts, half a cup

For the optional cream cheese frosting:
- 4 ounces (1/2 cup) softened cream cheese
- 1 1/2 cups of powdered sugar, 1/4 cup softened unsalted butter.
- Vanilla extract, 1/2 teaspoon.

Directions:

Turn on the oven to 350 °F (175 °C). Paper liners or cooking spray may be used to gently oil a muffin pan.

Mix the flour, baking powder, baking soda, salt, cinnamon, nutmeg, ginger and cloves in a medium bowl. Discard this dry mixture.

It should take around 2-3 minutes to beat the softened butter and granulated sugar together in a large mixing bowl until it becomes light and fluffy.

One at a time, beat in the eggs, making sure each is well mixed before adding the next. Add the vanilla essence and stir.

Mix just till mixed after gradually incorporating the dry ingredients into the wet ones. Make sure not to overmix; a few lumps are OK.

To the muffin batter, stir in the shredded carrots and chopped walnuts.

Divide the batter evenly among the muffin cups, filling each approximately 2/3 full, using a spoon or an ice cream scoop.

A toothpick put into the centre of a muffin should come out clean after 20 to 25 minutes of baking in a preheated oven.

You may make the cream cheese icing *(if wanted)* while the muffins bake. Cream the softened cream cheese, butter, powdered sugar and vanilla extract in a separate dish until it is smooth and creamy.

After the muffins have finished baking, take them out of the oven and let them cool in the pan for a while. After that, move them to a wire rack to finish cooling.

Before piping or spreading cream cheese icing on top of the muffins, wait until they have cooled.

The handmade spiced carrot and walnut muffins are delicious, also warm spices, sweet carrots and crunchy walnuts make for a delicious mix in these muffins. They are the ideal snack or morning treat, whether you want to eat them with or without cream cheese icing.

Chapter 7: Meal Plans and Tips

Weekly Meal Plans

Beginner's Week:

A wonderful method to begin eating better and cooking at home is to create a beginner's weekly meal plan. Here is a straightforward menu plan for a week, including ideas for breakfast, lunch and supper.

Depending on your dietary choices and needs, feel free to modify the portion proportions and the components. Drink water throughout the day to keep hydrated and if you are hungry in between meals, think about reaching for some fruit or nuts as a nutritious snack.

Day 1:

Breakfast:
- Scrambled eggs with tomatoes and spinach
- Whole grain bread
- Citrus juice

Lunch:

- Salad with grilled chicken breast, cherry tomatoes and balsamic vinaigrette.
- Whole-wheat roll

Dinner:

- Salmon baked with dill and lemon.
- Boiling broccoli
- Quinoa

Day 2:

Breakfast:

- Greek yoghurt, honey and a variety of fruit
- Granola with whole grains

Lunch:

- A wrap made with a whole-grain tortilla with turkey.
- Sticks of carrot and hummus

Dinner:

- Teriyaki sauce, mixed veggies and tofu in a stir-fry
- Dark rice

Day 3:

Breakfast:
- Sliced bananas and cinnamon sprinkled on top of muesli
- Nutella milk

Lunch:
- Chicken breast filled with spinach and feta
- Sweet potatoes roasted
- Green beans steamed

Dinner:
- Whole-grain pasta with marinara sauce for spaghetti with Italian dressing as a side salad.

Day 4:

Breakfast:
- Fresh strawberries on whole-grain waffles with a dollop of Greek yoghurt

Lunch:
- Corn, red pepper and lime vinaigrette on top of a quinoa and black bean salad
- Wheat-based crackers

Dinner:
- Garlic and herb-infused grilled prawn skewers
- Cooked asparagus
- Couscous

Day 5:

Breakfast:
- Blend bananas, peanut butter and almond milk to make a smoothie.

Lunch:
- Sandwich made with whole-grain bread and tuna salad
- Young carrots

Dinner:
- Baked chicken thighs with garlic and rosemary
- Chopped cauliflower

- Boiled broccoli

Day 6:

Breakfast:
- Bell peppers, onions and spinach in a veggie omelette
- Whole grain bread

Lunch:
- Bean soup
- Vinaigrette-dressed salad with mixed greens

Dinner:
- Baked cod with lemon and herbs
- Quinoa
- Sauteing asparagus

Day 7:

Breakfast:
- Overnight oats with almond milk, chia seeds and mixed fruit

Lunch:
- Fresh mozzarella, tomatoes and basil in a caprese salad with balsamic sauce.

Dinner:
- Stir-fry with grilled vegetables and chickpeas
- Dark rice

To reach your nutritional objectives, don't forget to drink lots of water throughout the day and modify portion sizes.

You may combine and change the meals in this meal plan to fit your tastes and dietary requirements. If you feel hungry in between meals, take into account nutritious snacks like yoghurt, fruits or almonds.

Weight Management Plan:

To reach and maintain a healthy weight, you need a weight-management strategy. It calls for a mix of healthy eating, consistent exercise and lifestyle adjustments. Here is a food plan and advice to assist you in managing your weight:

1. Set realistic objectives

Prior to beginning any weight-loss programme, be sure your objectives are doable. Instead of looking for fast remedies, focus on sustained, steady weight reduction or maintenance.

2. Diet that is balanced

Ensure that your diet is well-balanced and contains a selection of items from each dietary category. You will get important nutrients as a result.

- Include lean protein sources in your meals, such as chicken, turkey, fish, tofu and beans.

- For fibre, vitamins and minerals, consume a lot of fruits and vegetables.

- Select whole grains over refined grains, such as brown rice, quinoa and whole wheat bread.

- Reduce the amount of processed meals, sweetened beverages and high-calorie snacks you consume.

3. Portion Management

Be mindful of portion sizes. To regulate portion proportions, use measuring cups, a food scale or your palm as a guide.

In restaurants, try to order smaller servings and think about splitting meals or bringing half home.

4. Routine Meals

Throughout the day, have frequent, well-balanced meals to avoid severe hunger and subsequent overeating.

5. Intentional Eating

By focusing on the flavour, texture, and enjoyment of each mouthful, practise mindful eating. While eating, stay away from distractions like TV and cell phones.

Eat mindfully and quit when you are full but not stuffed.

6. Keep Hydrated

Drink a lot of water all day long. Sometimes, hunger and thirst are confused.

7. Nutritious Snacks

If you need a snack in between meals, choose healthy options like yoghurt, almonds, fruits or veggies.

8. Make a Meal Plan

Make a plan for your meals and snacks. You can do this to make better decisions and prevent impulsive, unhealthy eating.

9. Consistent Exercise

Make regular exercise a part of your regimen. Aim to do at least twice a week of strength training exercises together with at least 150 minutes of moderate-intensity aerobic activity or 75 minutes of intense activity each week.

10. Get Enough Sleep

Hormones that control appetite may be disturbed by sleep deprivation, which can result in overeating. Attempt to get 7-9 hours of restful sleep each night.

11. Stress reduction

Find healthy coping mechanisms for stress, such as deep breathing exercises, yoga or meditation. Emotional eating and stress go hand in hand.

12. Seek Support:

To help you remain on track and achieve your objectives, think about joining a support group or working with a healthcare expert, such a certified dietitian or personal trainer.

Do note that managing your weight is a long-term commitment. Be kind to yourself and implement long-lasting adjustments that you can keep up over time.

Gut Reset Challenge:

A gut reset challenge might be a terrific approach to enhance your general well-being and digestive health. You may finish the gut reset challenge with the aid of the following food plans and advice:

Remove Trigger Foods in Week 1

Focus on removing items that have a reputation for causing stomach irritation throughout the first week of your gut reset challenge. These may consist of:

Avoid processed foods that are heavy in refined grains, added sugars and artificial additives.

Eliminate gluten by avoiding foods made of wheat, such as bread, pasta and baked goods.

Dairy: Since many individuals are lactose intolerant or sensitive to dairy, avoid milk, cheese and yoghurt.

Highly processed oils should be avoided in favour of more healthful fats like coconut oil or olive oil.

Reduce or completely avoid your use of alcohol and caffeine.

Plan your meals:

Breakfast: A spinach, banana, almond milk, and protein powder smoothie.

Lunch would be a salad of grilled chicken or tofu with mixed greens, avocado and a simple dressing of olive oil and lemon.

Snack: A variety of nuts and seeds.

Dinner will consist of quinoa, steamed veggies and baked salmon or a plant-based protein source.

Tips:

Throughout the day, drink a lot of water to stay hydrated. To encourage a healthy gut microbiota, include fermented foods like kefir, kimchi and sauerkraut in your diet.

To help with digestion, chew your meal completely.

Reintroduce Gut-Friendly Foods Week 2

Reintroduce gut-friendly foods that support a healthy microbiome gradually throughout the second week:

Foods High in Fibre: Eat a lot of fruits, vegetables, and whole grains like quinoa, brown rice and oats.

Yoghurt, kefir, kombucha and fermented vegetables are all probiotic-rich foods that you should include in your diet.

Consider using bone broth in your meals since it is full of minerals that are good for the intestines.

Drink herbal teas to calm your digestive tract, such as chamomile, ginger and peppermint.

Plan your meals:

Breakfast will consist of overnight oats, yoghurt, and a variety of berries.

Lunch: Brown rice and a vegetable stir-fry with tofu or another low protein for lunch.

Snack: Greek yoghurt with honey and chia seeds as a snack.

Dinner will be baked fish or chicken with steamed vegetables and bone broth.

Tips:

As you reintroduce meals, pay attention to how your body is responding.

Increase fibre consumption gradually to avoid bloating or discomfort.

Drink plenty of water.

Week 3: Continue and Check

You need to have a better idea of how your digestive system responds to various meals by the third week. Maintain a healthy diet that is balanced and full of items that are good for your stomach. Pay attention to any particular meals that can cause pain or gastrointestinal problems.

Plan your meals:

Maintain your fibre, probiotic and lean protein-rich diet. Your meals should include a diversity of fruit and vegetable colours.

Maintain a regular eating schedule and stay hydrated.

Tips:

To keep track of your meals and any digestive issues, keep a food diary.

As stress may damage gut health, try stress-reduction tactics like deep breathing or meditation.

If you have ongoing digestive problems or worries, speak with a medical expert.

Remember that every individual has a different gut, so what works for one person may not work for another. Throughout the gut reset challenge, be patient and aware of your body's cues. If you have any underlying digestive issues or concerns, speak with a doctor.

Tips for Dining Out, Staying Consistent and Building Healthy Habits

Even though eating out while attempting to stick to a healthy diet might be difficult, you can choose healthy foods with little forethought and attention. Some pointers for eating out, maintaining your healthy eating routines and developing a long-term nutritional strategy:

1. Do Some Advance Menu Research:

Nowadays, a lot of eateries provide their menus online. Utilise this time to check the menu and decide on a healthier food before you arrive.

2. Seek out Healthy Alternatives:

Look for meals that contain veggies, nutritious grains, and lean meats like chicken, fish or tofu.

Avoid fried or sautéed foods in favour of grilled, baked or steamed alternatives.

3. Consider Portion Sizes:

Frequently, restaurant servings are bigger than you really need. If you want to divide the lunch in half, think about sharing it with a buddy or getting a to-go box straight soon.

4. Pay Attention to Beverages:

Instead of consuming sugary sodas or alcoholic beverages, go for water, herbal tea or other calorie-free liquids.

If you do consume alcohol, do it sparingly and be mindful of the additional calories it may include.

5. Make Your Order Custom:

Never be hesitant to request changes, such as more veggies in place of fries or sauce or dressing on the side.

6. Use Caution When Choosing Sides and Appetisers:

Side dishes and appetisers may have a lot of calories. If you want an appetiser, think of a vegetable-based dish or a salad.

Replace harmful sides like fries with steamed veggies or a side salad.

7. Put Portion Control to Use:

To determine portion amounts, use visual indicators like your hand. A portion of protein, for instance, should be around the size of your hand.

8. Mindful Eating:

Enjoy your meal slowly and mindfully. This may assist you in identifying fullness and preventing overeating.

9. Steer clear of unlimited buffets:

Buffets may promote binge eating. If you do eat at a buffet, concentrate on modest quantities and pile salads and vegetables on your plate.

10. Eat a full meal before going out to eat:

Overeating might result from skipping meals in anticipation of eating out. Early in the day, have a small, healthy meal or snack.

11. Maintain Consistency:

Attempt to adhere as closely as possible to your usual eating routine, especially while dining out. Healthy behaviours must be maintained consistently.

12. Plan Treat Meals:

When eating out, give yourself the occasional treat, but make sure it was a deliberate decision and not an impulse.

13. Track Your Food

To keep track of your meals, particularly when you eat out, think about using a food diary or a smartphone app. You can maintain accountability by doing this.

14. Exercise Moderation Rather Than Deprivation:

It's OK to sometimes indulge in unhealthy cuisine. Instead of rigorous deprivation, aim for balance and moderation.

15. Stay Active:

Include regular exercise in your daily routine to help balance out any odd excesses.

Establishing and sustaining good eating habits takes time. If you periodically stray from your plan when eating out, don't be too harsh on yourself. Recovering and continuing to make healthy decisions the majority of the time is crucial.

Chapter 8: Resources

Grocery Shopping List

Kitchen Equipment Checklist:

Meal planning and using the proper cooking tools may make home cooking more effective and pleasurable. Here is a list of kitchen supplies, as well as some sites for menu planning and culinary advice:

Checklist for Kitchen Appliances

Cookware:

- Nonstick and stainless steel skillets
- Pots and saucepans of different sizes
- French oven
- Baking pans and sheets
- Cooking tin

Utensils:

- Kitchen knife
- Chopping block
- Chopping block
- Mixing vessels
- Wooden spatulas and spoons

- Tongs
- Whisk
- Open a can
- Measuring spoons and cups
- Colander/strainer

Appliances:
- Oven
- Stovetop
- Microwave
- Toasters or toasters
- A food processor or blender
- Simmering pot or Instant Pot
- Espresso machine or kettle

Bakeware:
- Cake dishes
- Cookie tin
- Bread pan
- Pie plate
- A rolling pin
- Parchment paper for baking
- Cookie trays

Small Devices:
- Oven and meat thermometer
- Peeler
- Grater
- Timer
- Cooking scale
- Storage receptacles
- Includes lids, plastic or glass containers
- Food wrappers that can be reused *(like beeswax wraps)*
- Cooking necessities
- Cooking oil *(vegetable and/or olive)*
- Pepper and salt
- Herbs & spices
- *(Homemade or canned)* Stock or broth
- Vinegar *(such as apple cider, white and balsamic)*

Cleaning Products:

Hand soap

A drying mat or dish rack

Scrubbers or sponges

Containers for recycling and trash

Resources for Meal Preparation and Cooking Advice

Apps for meal planning: It's simple to plan and organise your meals with the help of meal planning apps like Mealime, Plan to Eat and Paprika.

Websites and blogs about cooking: A variety of recipes and culinary advice may be found on websites like AllRecipes, Food Network and culinary Light.

For in-depth recipe guides and culinary guidance, check out sites like Smitten culinary, Serious Eats and The Kitchn.

Cookbooks: Numerous cookbooks exist that cater to different cuisines and nutritional needs. Find those that fit your interests and degree of expertise.

Channels on YouTube: There are many culinary lessons on YouTube. Cooking instructions and step-by-step directions may be found on channels like Tasty, Bon Appétit and Jamie Oliver.

Templates for meal planning: To help you organise your weekly meals and grocery lists, you may find downloadable meal planning templates online.

Classes in cooking: To develop your culinary abilities, think about enrolling in live or online cooking lessons.

On social media: For recipe ideas and culinary advice, follow chefs, food bloggers and other cooking lovers on social media sites like Instagram and Pinterest.

Workshops for local chefs: Check to see if there are any local culinary courses or programmes where you may pick up practical knowledge and skills.

Note that based on your culinary tastes and style, you could require different tools and materials. Make sure your kitchen has the tools and resources you need for the meals you want to cook.

Conclusion:

Your Journey to a Healthy Colon

Keeping your colon in good shape is crucial for general health and may help avoid a number of gastrointestinal problems, including colorectal cancer. A path to a healthy colon via dietary choices and preventative actions is provided here:

Healthy Eating:

Eat a lot of fruits, vegetables, whole grains, and legumes to increase your intake of high-fibre foods. Due to the high fibre content of these meals, regular bowel movements are encouraged and constipation is avoided.

Limit Red Meat: Red and processed meats have been associated with an increased risk of colon cancer, so cut down on your intake of both.

Keep Hydrated: To keep your digestive system running smoothly, drink lots of water.

Exercise on a regular basis: On most days of the week, try to get in at least 30 minutes of moderate activity. Regular exercise may support good digestion and help you maintain a healthy weight.

Don't Drink Too Much and Don't Smoke: Smoking and excessive alcohol intake both raise the risk of colorectal cancer. To protect your colon, limit or stay away from these chemicals.

Screening for colon cancer: Follow your doctor's advice for screening for colon cancer, which may involve stool tests, sigmoidoscopies or colonoscopies. If cancer is present, early identification may result in improved results.

Keeping a Healthy Weight in Mind

Colon cancer risk factors include obesity. By eating a balanced diet and getting regular exercise, try to reach and maintain a healthy weight.

Eat less processed foods: High concentrations of harmful fats, carbohydrates and additives are often found in processed meals. Limit the amount of processed and quick food you eat.

Control Stress: Your digestive system may be impacted by ongoing stress. Use stress-relieving methods like yoga, meditation or deep breathing exercises and water consumption is important for healthy digestion and general well being. Aim for 8 to 10 glasses of water every day, minimum.

Reduce Your Antibiotic Use: Antibiotic overuse may alter the balance of healthy microorganisms in your stomach. Only take antibiotics as directed by a doctor and be sure you follow all of their recommendations.

Recognise Your Family's Past: Talk to your healthcare professional if you have a family history of colorectal cancer or other gastrointestinal problems. They could advise more frequent or earlier tests.

Stay Up to Date: Keep abreast on new discoveries in the fields of colon health, cancer prevention and medical science.

Genetics may also affect colon health, so it's mandatory to speak with a medical expert for personalised guidance and regular check-ups. You may lower your risk of colon-related problems and experience greater overall well-being by leading a healthy lifestyle and taking an active approach to colon health.

Embracing the Colon Diet Lifestyle And Transforming Your Health, One Recipe at a Time

A balanced diet consists of fruits, vegetables, whole grains, lean meats and healthy fats to provide optimum health.

Consuming fibre-rich meals helps maintain a healthy digestive system and regular bowel movements. Drinking enough water is crucial for digestion and overall health.

Limiting processed foods, which often contain harmful fats, excessive sugar and additives, can enhance health alongside controlling portion sizes, this can help manage weight and avoid overeating.

Mindful eating can help make healthy decisions and avoid thoughtless or emotional eating. Customising your eating plan to meet your unique nutritional needs can be done by consulting a healthcare expert or registered dietitian.

Regular physical exercise is essential for general health and can enhance a balanced diet. Consult a healthcare professional before making significant dietary changes, especially if you have specific health issues or ailments.

Enjoy Delicious Meals & Stay Healthy.